Self-Organizing Systems
The Long View
Your 27th Psychiatric Consultation
William R. Yee M.D., J.D.,
Copyright Applied for May 27th, 2021

The practice of medicine and psychiatry has been changing for many thousands of years.

Since 1972 the rate of change has been exponential and as unpredictable as the weather and the stock market.

Life in general is as unpredictable as the weather and the stock market.

Initially, religion, and superstition guided the practice of psychiatry and medicine.

The scientific method emerged as the tool that guided the progress of medicine.

Chaos Theory emerged as the best model for predicting the weather, the stock market, and social organizations such as medical organizations and the insurance industry.

The central fact of Chaos Theory is that short term predictions can be accurate, but long-term predictions cannot be accurate.

Another central fact is that although self-organizing systems may have the same starting rules, they can be very different in appearance and function due to small variations in starting points.

Human beings have about 99.4% identical DNA.

However, human beings also have 0.6% variation in DNA.

That means that all self-organizing social systems have slight differences in starting points simply based upon DNA variance among its members.

Central agencies set the rules for self-organizing systems with the intent of achieving consistency in outcomes for the long term.

Chaos Theory and the mathematics of nonlinear functions intervene and disrupts long term consistency.

Central agencies must constantly struggle
with the long-term unpredictable nature
of Self Organizing Systems.

I rely on

Self-Organization in Social Groups. In:
Tschacher W., Schiepek G., Brunner E.J.
(eds) Self-Organization and Clinical
Psychology.
Tschacher W., Brunner E.J., Schiepek G.
(1992)
Springer Series in Synergetics, vol 58.
Springer, Berlin, Heidelberg.
https://doi.org/10.1007/978-3-642-77534-5_19

Minimalist Management and Money

People with a Master's Degree in Business
Administration, (MBAs) have dominated
all businesses in the United States and
worldwide for many decades.

Dr. Budd was the last psychiatrist who
was the CEO of any mental health facility
I worked for.

That was in Northville State Hospital 1974
and 1975.

The reason is the launch of MBA programs and minimalist management strategies.

Minimalist management is a strategy to minimize cost and maximize profits. MBA's hire the minimum number of people who are the least qualified at the lowest rate of pay to get the job done.

This strategy comes with many costs that will emerge throughout the rest of this missive.

Small differences in education, knowledge, and competence can have large effects on the operation of any organization.

It is cheaper to hire someone with less training than a psychiatrist to function as a CEO.

One cost is that the risks and benefits of psychiatric and medical interventions are not well understood by the non-medical CEO.

Costs and revenue streams take priority over safety and the welfare of the personnel and customer base.

The Central Agencies in Washington D.C, the state capitals, Silicon Valley and other locations are confronted with risk management in the context of the Butterfly Effect in Chaos Theory.

The Butterfly Effect is that a small difference today can have huge and unpredictable implications in the future.

Predatory business practices eventually are brought to the attention of juries and juries respond by granting huge awards as punitive damages.

I refer the reader to Grimshaw v. Ford Motor Company, 1981, as the poster child for the Butterfly Effect in managing risk

Ford Motor Company determined that it would be cheaper to pay damage awards for death than to install a $10 plate above the gas tank.

The actuaries calculated that the cost of installing the ten-dollar plate exceeded the cost of paying families for the deaths of the burned passengers in the Pinto cars.

The jury read the internal memos recommending against installing a metal plate between the gas tank and the passenger apartment of the Pinto automobile.

The jury awarded $2.516 million to the Grimshaws and $559,680 to the Grays in damages for their injuries. For good measure the jury added $125 million to punish Ford for its conduct.

That $125 million awarded in punitive damages was the jury's way of changing risk management in the automobile industry.

Let us examine the difficulty the government in Sacramento California has in managing costs in the prison system in California.

Vaughn Dorch was a prisoner in Pelican Bay Prison in Crescent City, California.

Pelican Bay Prison was a Maximum-Security Prison for isolating the most violent criminals from the general population and large urban centers in California.

Vaughn Dortch had a life-long history of mental problems but was confined to the Violent Control Unit of the SHU at Pelican Bay Prison after a conviction for grand theft.

The reader should be advised that the prison culture embraces the use of urine and feces for "gassing," prison guards and staff for the purposes of intimidation and retaliation.

Gassing is throwing urine, feces, and blood into the eyes, noses and mouths of prison guards and staff. It is a felony and prison employees have died from Hepatitis C and HIV after being gassed by prisoners.

Working in prisons is unsafe and unpleasant.

Prisoners will smear their cells and themselves with urine and feces knowing that the prison guards must clean up the mess.

It was alleged that the stark conditions of isolation in Pelican Bay Prison caused Mr. Dortch's mental condition to deteriorate to the point that he smeared himself repeatedly with feces and urine. Smearing feces was also, however, prison culture.

Regardless of the reason, Mr. Dortch had a pattern of smearing himself and his cell with feces, which forced the prison employees to clean both Mr. Dortch and his cell.

Given the prison culture, this pattern of behavior could be considered a form of aggression on Mr. Dortch's part, rather than a symptom of mental illness.

In April 1992 prison officials, (the Warden?) ordered a bath.

Prison staff took Vaughn Dortch to the infirmary to bathe him.

When Mr. Dortch refused, prison guards forced him into a tub with hot water, resulting in burns to the lower parts of his body.

Neither the Warden nor the prison guards wanted to injure Mr. Dortch severely enough to require hospital treatment.

The Butterfly Effect and Murphy's Law manifested at this point. When Mr. Dortch stood up his skin fell off in sheets.

Mr. Dortch was taken to the hospital.

The hospital took photographs of the injuries.

At trial, the photographs were introduced as evidence.

When the photographs were introduced as evidence, they became part of a public record and were no longer protected medical records.

These pictures were then released to the public and placed onto the internet.

Mr. Vaughn Dortch filed sued and the case was settled, resulting in a payment of $997,000 to Dortch.

The judge ordered that the settlement be confidential, but 60 Minutes revealed the details on February 27, 1994.

The details were recounted by the lead prison nurse in the Madrid v. Gomez case that followed. See Madrid v. Gomez, 889 F.

Supp. 1146 (N.D. Cal. 1995). U.S. District Court for the Northern District of California - 889 F. Supp. 1146 (N.D. Cal. 1995) January 10, 1995

The bully? Mr. Dortch,? Prison employees? Both?

That is the question.

We have all been bullied on the playground of life.

Everyone has been bullied in the economic playground

Multinational corporations are viewed as the big bullies by most people that become jurors at trials.

Let us explore power and bullies that we meet on the playground through the lens of Self Organizing Systems.

Chaos Theory and Self Organizing Systems are the subject of a great deal of research based upon the mathematics of non-linear functions and simple rules of organization. Let us explore Power through this lens.

Power and Self Organizing Systems

The U.S. Office of Naval Research funded the Stanford Prison Experiment (SPE) to identify the root causes of difficulties between guards and prisoners in the United States Navy and United States Marine Corps.

The basic story is that the professor recruited students to be either guards or prisoners in a psychological laboratory on a college campus.

The students were healthy, intelligent, and educated without significant mental illness or prior history of violence or cruelty.

The Butterfly Effect and Murphy's Law intervened in a most unexpected way.

The experiment was stopped when the guards became cruel and ethical considerations compelled the professor to stop the experiment.

This was an unexpected outcome. Normal, healthy educated people become cruel simply because they had power over others.

Power Corrupts and Absolute Power
Corrupts Absolutely.

This thought was not a stranger to the
authors of the Constitution of the United
States. The entire constitution is designed
to prevent power from being concentrated
among a few individuals.

Divisions in government and frequent
elections all blunt opportunities to
centralize power.

I refer the reader to Philip Zimbardo who
is best-known for his 1971 Stanford Prison
Experiment which is described above.

Power corrupts and absolute power
corrupts absolutely is Old Wisdom that
has stood The Test of Time.

Democide is the murder of any person or
people by their government, including
genocide, politicide, and mass murder.

Democide causes more deaths than war.

Rudolph Rummel estimated 262 million
victims of democide in the last century.

Wikipedia has more information for the interested reader, including references.

The Stockholm Syndrome

The Stockholm Syndrome manifests when hostages, or abuse victims, bond with their captors or abusers.

The most famous case was Patty Hearst.

Patricia Campbell Hearst born February 20, 1954, was a granddaughter of American publishing magnate William Randolph Hears.

Patty Hearst was kidnapped by the Symbionese Liberation Army in 1974.

Patty Hearst was caught on camera assisting the Symbionese Liberation Army in a bank robbery.

Patty Hearst asserted that she was raped and threatened with death and forced to take part in the bank robbery.

She was convicted and then pardoned.

The Stockholm Syndrome is still alive and well in the scientific literature and jury trials are fascinating studies of how a jury of twelve responds to the experts and legal arguments.

The police officer dreads domestic violence calls for good reason. Domestic violence calls often result in an officer shot or killed.

Occasionally the victim will assault the arresting officer resulting in the death of the police officer. This is The Stockholm Syndrome through the lens of a police officer.

The social worker, psychiatrist, and Child Protective Services all wrestle with the Stockholm Syndrome at their own peril.

The Compliance Agreement

In 1987 I interviewed for the position of Director of Mental Health Services for the Michigan Department of corrections.

The director of health care for the Michigan Department of Corrections would be a Psychiatrist VII position. That was the highest possible civil service ranking in 1987.

I was board certified in psychiatry, I was licensed to practice law, and I had been the Chairman of the Department of Psychiatry at a community hospital. I also had more than two years of experience as a Medical Director of a four-county mental health center in Indiana.

The first interview went well.

Murphy's Law intervened and changed the course of my life.

Murphy's Law Shocks the Conscience

Murphy's Law, if something can go wrong, eventually it will go wrong.

I was invited back for a second interview with the expectation that I would be offered the position of Director of Mental Health Services for the Department of Correctios for the State of Michigan.

When I arrived, I was told that the person who interviewed me was no longer working for the Michigan Department of Corrections.

That was unexpected.

The Michigan Department of Corrections was under the supervision of the Federal Courts for violating the constitutional standard of care for the mentally ill prisoners.

At that time three out of four state hospitals and prisons were under the supervision of the federal courts for violating the prisoners' rights to basic health care.

The reader needs to understand the different standards of care.

The highest standard of care is the standard of care of a specialist, such as a psychiatrist, heart surgeon, pediatrician, or Obstetrician/Gynecologist.

The specialist practices under a national standard of care and a specialist from anywhere in the country can be called in to testify as to the standard of care for that specialty.

A lower standard of care is the standard of care provided by a general practitioner.

The general practitioner practices under a local standard of care and general practitioners in that neighborhood may be called in to testify as to what the local standard of care is for that neighborhood.

The Constitutional Standard of Care for the mentally ill in jails, prisons, and state hospitals is, "shocks the conscience."

This is the lowest possible standard of care and is often litigated.

That is why three out of four State hospitals and prisons were under the supervision of the federal courts.

Most prisons and state hospitals were providing such poor care that juries made a finding of fact that the care shocked the conscience. The state prisons and state hospital were then put under the supervision of the federal courts for corrective actions.

When I returned to accept the position as Director of Mental Health Services for the Michigan Department of Corrections, my supervisor was no longer there to hire me. He had signed a Compliance Agreement with the Federal Courts to improve services for the mentally ill prisoners. The Michigan Department of Corrections did not like the Compliance Agreement and fired him before I was hired.

As the Medical Director for Mental Health Services for the Michigan Department of Corrections I would have had the pay and benefits of a Psychiatrist VII in Civil Service.

I was supporting a family and in need of employment. I took a job as line staff, a psychiatrist III.

I was going to do direct patient care at Riverside Psychiatric Hospital in Ionia, Michigan. This was a psychiatric hospital operated by the Michigan Department of Corrections. The warden was a clinical psychologist charged with managing violence in the Michigan Department of Corrections.

Managing Violent Prisoners

In November of 1987 I entered Riverside Psychiatric Hospital as a Psychiatrist III.

Riverside Psychiatric Hospital was an
experiment in managing violence in the
Michigan Department of Corrections.

At that time prison wardens were
responsible for injuries to correctional
officers and prisoners.

At that time prison wardens were
authorized to label violent prisoners as
mentally ill and transfer them to
Riverside Psychiatric Hospital in Ionia,
Michigan.

As a result, Riverside Psychiatric Hospital
housed one hundred violent prisoners.

Riverside Psychiatric Hospital had an
average of about 5.2 workmen
compensation cases per month due to
assaults resulting in injuries severe
enough to result in time off from work.

I arrived for my first day of duty on
Monday, November 16th, 1987.

Riverside Psychiatric Hospital was a
prison hospital surrounded by razor wire.

The building was a two-story building
with two twenty-five bed units on the

ground floor and two twenty-five bed units on the second floor.

There were supposed to be two psychiatrists for each unit with a case load of twelve or thirteen patients for each psychiatrist.

I was the fourth psychiatrist and was awarded a full twenty-five bed unit all to myself.

On Tuesday, December the 1st, 1987 I arrived at work at eight o'clock in the morning and was told that I was now in charge of the entire Riverside Psychiatric Hospital as the other three psychiatrists took, vacation or medical leave for the entire month.

I spent the rest of the day and the entire month doing restraints and medication reviews with little time for talking to the patients.

The reader can decide whether this was Murphy's Law come to roost, or Minimalist Management and MBAs at their best. Perhaps both?

I will say that I worked at Riverside Psychiatric Hospital from November of 1987 to July of 1991.

From November of 1987 to July 1981, I saw a parade of psychiatrists interviewing for the empty positions.

However, there were never more than four psychiatrists on duty at any given time that I can recall.

Was the policy to interview and not hire?

Was this Minimalist Management hard at work?

Does this shock the conscience?

I leave it to the reader to research the facts and make an educated guess.

I suggest George Carlin and W. C. Fields for appropriate commentary on the marriage of Minimalist Management and Government.

The weakness is the fact that there are governmental immunities against lawsuits and the Chain of Command in

Civil Service are usually not held accountable for their errors.

The state pays for the damages and the Chain of Command continues without punishment or motivation to change the culture.

Antisocial Personalities and Prisons

Antisocial Personalities are often portrayed as living well off the suffering of others.

This may be true outside of prison.

However, in prison, antisocial personalities are often unhappy and at an elevated risk for suicide.

About a third of prisoners in the United States are antisocial personality disorders.

For additional information and a bibliography for research I refer the reader to:

Antisocial personality disorder in incarcerated offenders: Psychiatric comorbidity and quality of life

Donald W Black 1, Tracy Gunter, Peggy Loveless, Jeff Allen, Bruce Sieleni
Ann Clin Psychiatry. 2010 May;22(2):113-20.
PMID: 20445838

Since 1987 I have treated prisoners in Riverside Psychiatric Hospital, Bellamy Creek, I-Max, Brooks, Muskegon, Michigan Reformatory, Richard A. Handlon Correctional Facility in Michigan.

Since 2011 I have treated prisoners in California State Prison Sacramento, Pelican Bay State Prison, and San Quentin State Prison.

Antisocial Personalities
The Good, Bad, & Ugly

At Riverside psychiatric hospital the prisoner with the most violent reputation was the most puzzling. He knocked out an entire squad who rushed his room in body armor.

He was always polite and respectful when I talked to him.

He did not present with significant mental illness.

Our conversations were always pleasant. I advised him that he had good parents because his social skills were excellent.

I asked him how he came to have such a bad reputation for violence and why he was not violent during my time with him.

His answer was simple and direct.

""I just got tired of fighting."

Antisocial Personality Disorder will remit at mean age of 35 years at a rate of 12 to 27% and 27 to 31% rates of improvement.

For more information and bibliographies for additional research I refer the reader to the following:

Antisocial Personality Disorder
Kristy A. Fisher; Manassa Hany.
Treasure Island (FL): StatPearls
Publishing; 2021 Jan-.

and

Age and remission of psychiatric
disorders
R C Bland 1, S C Newman, H Orn
Can J Psychiatry. 1997 Sep;42(7):722-9.
doi: 10.1177/070674379704200704.
PMID: 9307832
DOI: al 10.1177/070674379704200704

Unexpected Consequences

The Dortch case above is the best example
of unexpected consequences. When there
is a chain of command in the state capital
and state hospitals or prisons at many
distant sites there are infinite
possibilities of unintended consequences.

Social Engineering

Social Engineering is popular among
diverse groups and special interests.

Social Engineering has resulted in many
identified protected minorities and many
laws that give the protected minorities
rights including special accommodations
which the average person is not entitled
to.

Handicapped parking spaces are the most common and easily identified right for protected minorities.

Let us look at social engineering for the purpose of giving females equal rights to work and equal pay. In the 1980's women started working as correctional officers in the Michigan state prisons

A union official in Ionia, Michigan made a statement that was published in the local newspaper.

He stated that the only reason a woman would work as a correctional officer in a prison was to find a man for a husband.

His public statement was unexpected by many.

Murphy's Law and the Butterfly effect intervened.

That union official was forced to resign.

He did not expect to be forced to resign because he merely voiced the consensus opinion of the correctional officers. His statement was most likely intended to improve his popularity and increase the probability of his reelection.

In 1987 one of the first female correctional officers started working at Jackson State Prison.

She was not on the job very long before she was murdered in the prison yard.

She was in a secluded place without line of sight by other correctional officers.

It was widely known that male correctional officers did not want women among their ranks because the males did not believe that females were physically capable of managing prisoners and would jeopardize the safety of the male correctional officers.

It was widely rumored that this female officer was set up to be murdered to discourage females from working as correctional officers.

The murder became a matter of national news and debate.

There were other issues including sexual harassment of female officers.

I rely on my direct observations and:

PRISON MURDER PROMPTS PROBE
CHICAGO TRIBUNE
August 2nd, 1987.

"Suicide by cop."
An FBI official acknowledged that the
bureau classified the mass shooting that
left a U.S. representative in perilous
condition and wounded several U.S.
Capitol Police officers as a "suicide by
cop."

Another major issue in controlling state
agencies is the accuracy of memory and
reports as to compliance with policies and
procedures.

Failure to comply with policies and
procedures is expected because memory
is reconstructed. The reconstruction of
memories results in predictable errors.

Truth is an imaginary construct.
Everyone knows what it is and no one has
bumped into it. Memories are
reconstructed constructs, and no two
people will describe the event the same

way as evidenced by conflicting stories
under oath

I rely on:

The fallibility of memory in judicial
processes:
Lessons from the past and their modern
consequences
Mark L. Howe, and Lauren M. Knott
Memory. 2015 Jul 4; 23(5): 633–656.
Published online 2015 Feb 23. doi:
10.1080/09658211.2015.1010709
PMCID: PMC4409058
PMID: 25706242

Another cause of errors in compliance
with policies and procedures are
structural and functional abnormalities in
the frontal lobe executive functions.

These abnormalities may be temporary
due to stress, anxiety or depression or
they may be permanent due to Attention
Deficit Disorder, Borderline Personality
Disorder, Traumatic Brain Injury, and
other causes.

Structural and Functional Brain
Abnormalities of the brain can be

identified by EEG's, CT scans, and fMRIs. The use of EEG's, CT scans and fMRIs to identify structural and functional abnormalities of the brain to guide diagnosis and treatment of mental illness is inevitable.

I refer the reader to:

Frontal Lobe Executive Function Dysfunction, Root Cause, The Long View Your 26th Psychiatric Consultation William R. Yee M.D., J.D Copyright Applied for May 24, 2021

I am here to do no harm and help if I can.

Thank you for your time and attention.

William R. Yee M.D., J.D.
Board Certified Psychiatrist.
Practicing Medicine and Psychiatry without interruption since 1972 in Michigan, Indiana, Kentucky, California and Texas at your service.

"Pre-Existing text," includes names of symptoms and medical illnesses, medications, people, corporations, law cases, statutes, text of statutes, the titles of articles and books, thecontent of articles and books cited, FDA Labels and FDA releases.

My copyright claim is a clam to the "original text," which is my personal experience as described in the text and my commentary on the names of symptoms and medical illnesses, medications, people, corporations, law cases, statutes, text of statutes, the titles of articles and books, the content of articles and books cited FDA Labels and FDA releases.

Ingram Content Group UK Ltd.
Milton Keynes UK
UKHW010022090623
423139UK00004B/45